The Teacher's Guide
To Less Stress!

A Quick & Easy Way to
Reduce Your Daily Stress

by

Carol L Rickard, LCSW
America's Ultimate Stress Expert

As Featured:

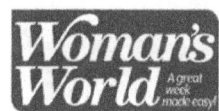

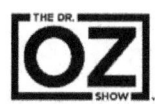

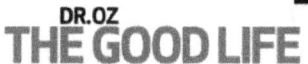

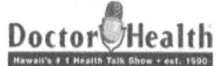

The Teacher's Guide to Less Stress
by Carol L Rickard, LCSW

© 2019 Carol L Rickard   All Rights Reserved

All rights reserved. No part of this book may be reproduced for resale, redistribution, or any other purposes (including but not limited to eBooks, pamphlets, articles, video or audiotapes, & handouts or slides for lectures or workshops). Permission to reproduce these materials for those and any other purposes must be obtained in writing from the author.

The author & publisher of this book do not dispense medical advice nor prescribe the use of this material as a form of treatment. The author & publisher are not engaged in rendering psychological, medical, or other professional services. The purpose of this material is educational only.

ISBN: 978-1-947745-15-5   (paperback)
ISBN: 978-1-947745-22-3   (Ebook)

Published by:

Well YOUniversity Publications
A Division of Well YOUniversity, LLC
5 Zion Rd.
Hopewell, NJ 08525
888 LIFE TOOLS (543-3866)
www.WellYOUniversity.com

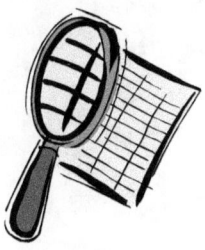

What will you get out of this book?

- A better understanding of WHY you must take action to reduce & manage your daily work stress.

- A simple & practical system that will decrease your STRESS levels in just 60 seconds or less!

- A long-lasting career you can now enjoy because you know how to *keep STRESS from ruining it!*

Table of Contents

Welcome	1
Getting Started	4
About this Book	10
What's The Impact	15
It's In the Cards	19
Tracking Progress	25

Part 1: Now You See It!

#1 – Root Beer	35
#2 – The Tub	44

Part 2: Now You Don't!

WHAT To Do	49
HOW To Do It - Step 1	57
HOW To Do It - Step 2	71

Part 3: A Solid Foundation!

Building a Solid Foundation	87
Wrap Up	115
DO*60* System *Mini Poster*	127
Keys to Success *Mini Poster*	129
The Stressometer™ *Mini Poster*	131
Carol's Other Resources	135

Sign Up For…

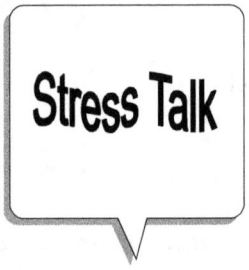

This 5-minute video newsletter will give you more tips, tools, & rules for taking control of…

STRESS!

Sign up at:

StressYOUniversity.com/Stress-Talk

Welcome

Stress comes wrapped up in

some pretty amazing packages…

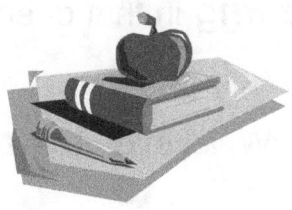

Your career happens to be one of them!

It's one of the **most fulfilling & special**

And yet

one of the **MOST** *stressful* as well!

If you are reading this  , there is

one thing I know for sure about you…

You are **either...**

at a breaking point

OR

heading in that direction.

Whichever it is –

I am glad you are here!

There is **NO** *shortage* when it comes to **work stress!**

From the education system & administration to students needs to parents and policies ...

There's plenty to go around & be shared.

The problem…

when **Stress** is not managed,

it has the *power to ruin* a lot of things…

health

    relationships

        hopes

           dreams

                &… careers.

It is my sincere hope you will take &

use what you learn in this book!

You will either manage your stress

or

IT CONTINUES TO MANAGE YOU!

Getting Started

Let me ask you a 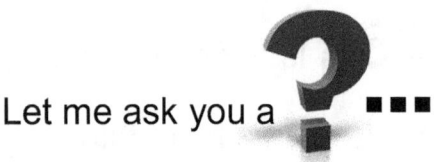...

What if you could learn how to

eliminate stress in just ***60 seconds***?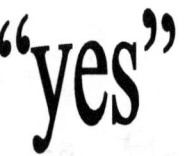

Would you want to know?

If the answer is **"yes"**

than just keep on reading!

You are about to learn a **revolutionary approach** to managing your stress.

This approach will put you in

control of stress once & for all.

It may seem like it is too good to be true –

But *it isn't!*

I'm going to share with you the

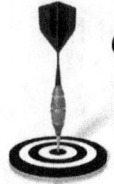 secret system I've been

teaching my patients since 1991.

Equally as important,

it is the same system I use every day…

I LIVE WHAT I TEACH!

That wasn't always the case…

When I started 17 years ago at the

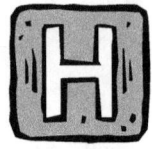

where I still currently work –

STRESS had *control* of me!

Only…

I didn't *realize* it…

It wasn't until I landed

in my doctor's office

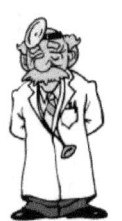

3 weeks in a row

with ***horrible migraines*** & he asked

"Carol, what's got you so stressed?"

Now, the most **embarrassing** part:

Here I was *teaching my patients*

the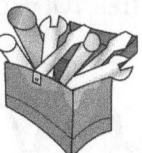

to manage their stress…

BUT I wasn't *using them myself!*

Since that day,

I have **kept** my commitment to

I LIVE WHAT I TEACH every day!

Everything I share here with you –

I use Myself!

My Biggest Excuse

I'd been in my new job at the hospital for about 8 months.

I LOVED IT!

In fact, I remember thinking to myself:

'I can't believe I am getting paid to do this!'

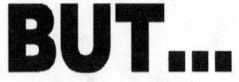

It was a busy place – so busy I didn't…

Get to stop & eat lunch

Get to take my breaks

Even step outside for 1 minute!

BUT…

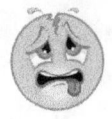 When the migraines hit me so HARD I knew I had to make a

Big change.

Leaving my job was not an option.

Besides –

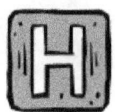 I knew from having worked at other hospitals, it would be the

same *STRESS everywhere.*

What had to **change was** **ME!**

I had to start using the tools I was teaching even if I only had *60* seconds.

That's how I *discovered my system works!*

About This Book

I doubt you have read a 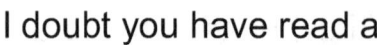 like this!

I like to use a lot of pictures, 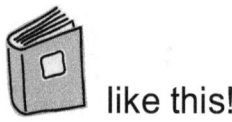 analogies, & word art which help information stick in the brain!

I call my approach:

SMARTheory™

(It's what makes my books and services *different* from all others!)

KNOWLEDGE is the *left brain* at work.

This is where YOU ***know*** what to do!

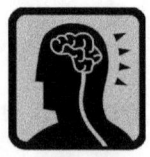

Since I use "pictures" & "images", I end up

tapping into the other side of the brain –

the right side!

With both sides working

on the same page,

the end result is getting people to

Move knowledge in to ACTION!

You'll find this book is broken in to 3 parts:

Part One: Now You See It!
Part Two: Now You Don't!
Part Three: A Solid Foundation

Part 1:

Here I introduce you to a concept

that will CHANGE

your life **forever**....

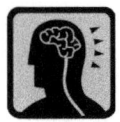 You'll never think about stress

the same way **again!**

You also learn WHY we must

DO **something about it.**

Did you know...

Studies show over 80% of people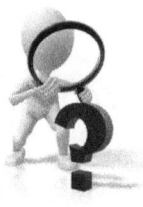

DO NOTHING about

their record high stress levels.

Part 2:

This section will ***give*** YOU the tools

to get the job done!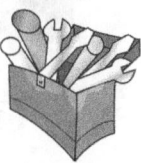

You'll learn **A LOT** of

different "tools"!

The secret I learned a long time ago…

Having the *right tool*

for the *right job* makes

the difference between

success and failure.

Also,
1 TOOL *won't work* the

same for everyone!

Part 3:

Stress has the power to

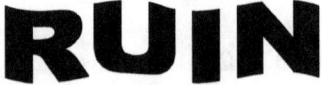

the BEST health.

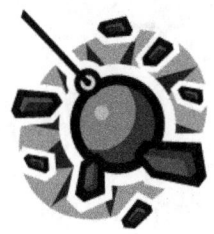

You're in **_even more_** trouble

if you're already having health issues.

We'll look at WHAT you

can do to make sure you

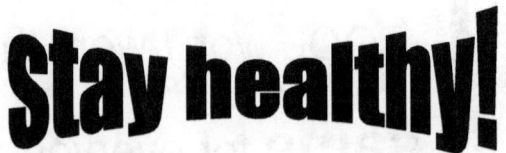

What's The Impact?

Stress can be found *all around the world*. Teachers are at ***epidemic*** levels - just look at some of the headlines:

The Graide NETWORK — SEPTEMBER 4, 2018

The Epidemic of Teacher Stress

MAY 11, 2018 · 1:02PM

neaToday

How Many Teachers Are Highly Stressed? Maybe More Than People Think.

BY TIM WALKER

K-12

Teachers Are Stressed, And That Should Stress Us All

December 30, 2016 · 4:59 AM ET
Heard on Morning Edition

US Population Statistics: (APA / AIS 7/28/14)

77%
Regularly experience physical symptoms caused by stress

54%
Say stress has caused them to fight with those they love.

76%
Identify money and work as the leading cause of stress

48%
Say stress has had a negative impact on their lives

$300 Billion
Estimated annual cost to US businesses / employers

So, what does this mean?

Stress is a... **HUGE** problem

The 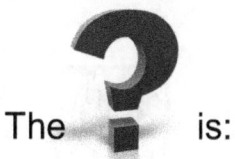 is:

What is stress COSTING YOU?

Are you so stressed out you can't sleep?

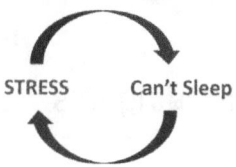

Is your stress spilling out on the wrong people or following you to work?

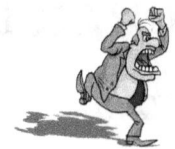
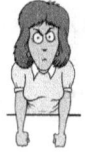

Is stress affecting your work?

Are you starting to have health issues?

 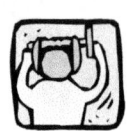 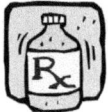

A "yes" to any of these is a sure sign **stress** has taken *CONTROL* of your life

There's **good** news!

You're reading this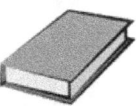

By the time you are finished…

You'll be able to **CONTROL IT** rather than *it controlling YOU!*

It's In The Cards!

When you come to my live seminars, as you take your seat, you'll be handed a playing card!

It may be a king, or it may be a three....

The **key point** is:

You **DON'T** get to **CHOOSE** what card you get!

This applies so wonderfully **to LIFE** – where we'll face many situations that

WE DON'T GET TO CHOOSE!

This is particularly the case

when you work in an education setting.

There are many days where you may

have a plan for how the day will go

and **it goes the other way.**

There are so many factors

you don't get to control…..

A student's behavior

Budgets

Administrators

Parents

Class Size

So,

what are you supposed to do?

All that you *can* do…

Play the cards you're dealt that day

the **BEST** that you can!

Here's a couple of the tools I've used:

It's not

WHAT HAPPENS

TO YOU,

BUT

HOW YOU REACT

TO IT

THAT MATTERS

EPICTETUS

Another way to think about it….

We don't get to control the events,

We *do get to control*

<u>our</u> <u>response</u> to them!

We are 100% responsible for our **choice:**

Controlling

How

Our

Intentions

Create

Experiences

© 2019 & licensed by Well YOUniversity, LLC

Taken from the *WordTools Series*

This is my favorite &

the *MOST* POWERFUL:

> WHEN WE FACE A SITUATION
>
> THAT *CANNOT* BE CHANGED
>
> WE ARE **CHALLENGED**
> TO
> *CHANGE OURSELVES*
>
> VICTOR FRANKL

Are you trying to change things

you CAN'T CONTROL?

Do the exercise on the next page to see!

Write down as many things you can think of having to do with teaching:

(Use another piece of paper if you need more room!)

Now go back & circle

ONLY the things **you can** control!

Tracking Your Progress

Monitoring

I developed a tool to help my patients be able to track their progress.

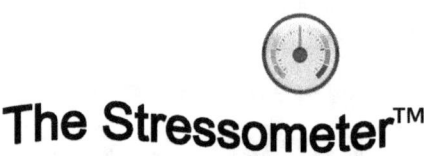

The Stressometer™

It's pretty simple to use!

1st - Read each question & select the answer that *best describes* you.

2nd - When you get to the end, *total up* all the numbers for a score

3rd - *Check your score* on the key. Repeat to see how you progress!

The Stressometer

I find when I try to go to sleep, my mind just keeps racing about things.

1	2	3	4	5	6	7
Not at all						All the time

I find my appetite changes, I'm either eating more or eating less.

1	2	3	4	5	6	7
Not at all						All the time

I find myself getting really angry over the littlest things.

1	2	3	4	5	6	7
Not at all						All the time

I find I am having increased health issues. (ie. migraines, pain, & digestive)

1	2	3	4	5	6	7
Not at all						All the time

I find my relationship is being impacted by what goes on at work / home.

1	2	3	4	5	6	7
Not at all						All the time

Total: _____

How Stressed Are You?

5–10 **Great news!**
> You have no stress!

11–15 **Good news!**
> You have just a little bit of stress!

16–20 **Not bad!**
> You seem to still have a handle on it!

21–25 **WATCH OUT!**
> STRESS is *starting to cause trouble!*

26–30 **WARNING…**
> STRESS is *greatly impacting* your life.

31–35 **DANGER Zone!**
> **Your level has you at extreme risk.**

Your score ***will come down*** when you use the system!!!

Another Tracking Tool

How to tell if this  is helping!

There are 2 more ways to track -

Both use a score of 1 to 100

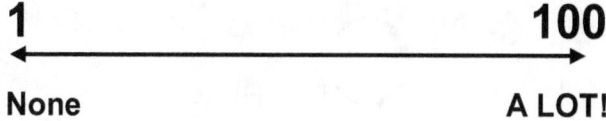

#1 Track your **daily** stress level
(do this every evening)

#2 Track your level **before & after** you use the tools!

**Since this is new for you
it may take a little time for you to
get used to the tools!**

For this system to WORK...

YOU must *take* **ACTION!**

Here are a couple of my **WordTools** to help:

A

Critical

Task

Implemented

Only

Now!

© 2019 & licensed by Well YOUniversity, LLC
Taken from the *WordTools Series*

No "tool" will work…

> if you don't **pick it up**
>
> &
>
> ***DO*** something with it!!

Here's my WordTool:

Direct

Opportunity

© 2019 & licensed by Well YOUniversity, LLC
Taken from the *WordTools Series*

Lastly,

When we **_DON'T_** use the "tools"

This is what happens!

Denied

Opportunity

Not

'

Trying

© 2019 & licensed by Well YOUniversity, LLC
Taken from the *WordTools Series*

Part One
Now You See It!
(Two ways to 'see' it!)

#1

Imagine this ...

I hand you a big bottle of root beer

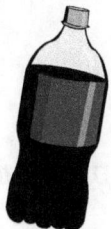

and ask you to *shake it up* –

A LOT!

Maybe you even **drop** it on the floor...

So, **what** do you think will **happen**

to the bottle of root beer?

You're **right!**

The PRESSURE builds up inside!

And once *the pressure gets built up*

It stays there...

It won't go away on its own.

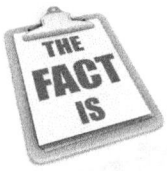

The PRESSURE doesn't go *anywhere*

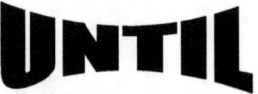

we *do something to let it out!*

And, it's *not good* to have **too much** PRESSURE build up inside the bottle.

Two things can happen…

#1 It comes SPILLING OUT & leaves a big mess.

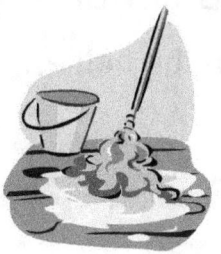

#2 It STAYS IN and ends up *ruining* the root beer.

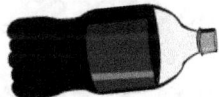

It's best to avoid both!

People are like the bottle ...

Things happen in life that

shake a person up

And…

　　Just like the pressure

　　BUILT UP

　　in the bottle…

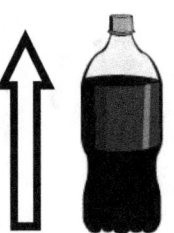

STRESS builds up *inside people!*

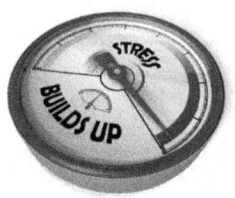

And once the *STRESS gets built up*

It stays there…

It won't go away on its own.

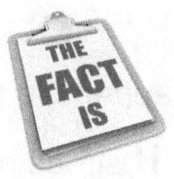

The **STRESS** doesn't go anywhere

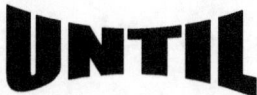

we *do something to let it out!*

(we'll talk about this in part 2)

And just like the bottle,

It's *not good* for **too much** STRESS to build up inside people!

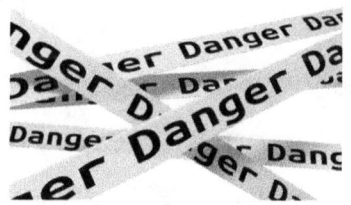

Here's what happens to people when **TOO MUCH** stress builds up…

#1 It comes SPILLING OUT & leaves a **big** mess.

Have you ever: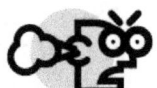

Said hurtful things or things you wished you hadn't said, yelled, got in arguments, broke things, had road rage, or slammed doors?

#2 It STAYS IN and ends up ruining *your health.*

Have you ever: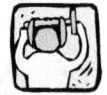

Felt anxiety, can't sleep, gotten headaches, ate too much or not at all, felt sad & depressed, couldn't concentrate, worried a lot?

Do any of the following everyday life things **STRESS** you out?

Chronic Pain

    Bills / Finances

        Looking for work

           Being a caregiver

                Dr's appointments

                  Holidays

Commute to work / school

    Relationships

        Not working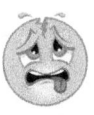

            Getting sick

                Family members

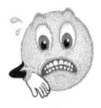   Kids / Pets

Running late or waking up late

 **Important news:**

A situation that *causes* one-person stress

may not *cause* you stress!

Now, what are the WORK things

stressing you out?

Write them down here:

(Use another piece of paper if you need more room!)

#2

What do you think would happen if…

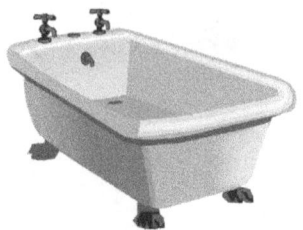

You *plugged* the drain,

turned the water **on**,

and then *walked away*?

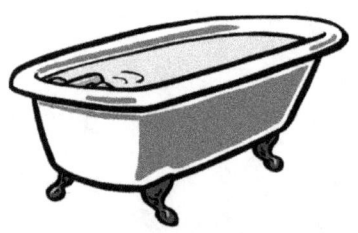

Eventually….

It would **overflow**, right?

Once it did – there'd be a

HUGE MESS!

Does this make sense?

A tub can only hold **so much!**

Two important points:

1) Once the level starts to rise – It will KEEP rising until it is **shut off.**

2) The tub ONLY has *so much room* - It can ONLY hold *so much* then it's

OVERFLOW!!!

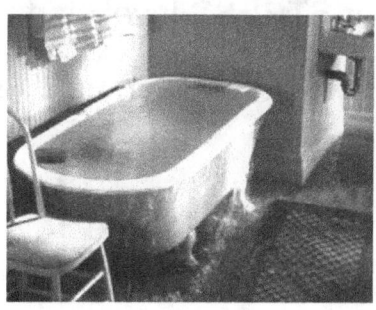

Some people think…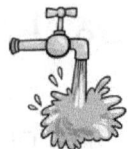

The solution is to just **turn OFF the water.**

You'll see later why this *won't* work!

When it comes to
STRESS…

People are just like a tub: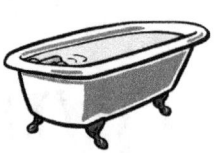

1) Once you wake up –

your **STRESS** level starts to rise

& it will keep rising until it is…

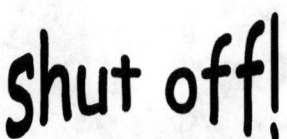

2) *YOU* only have *so much room* -

YOU can only hold so much

STRESS

until *YOU* will be at

OVERFLOW!!!

So,

I hope you can 👓 how

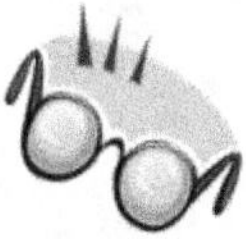

STRESS creates problems

And how it won't go away

until we…

release it!

Now that you can **SEE IT:**

Way #1

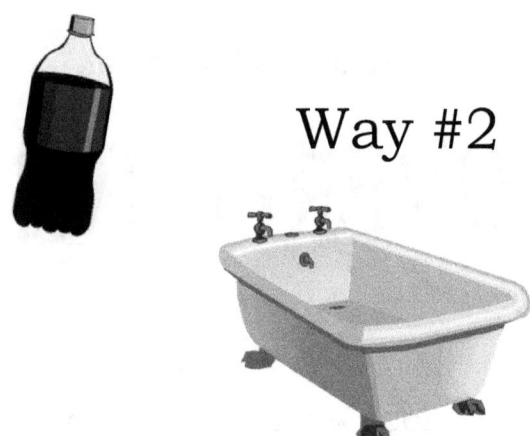

Way #2

It's time to learn how to

RELEASE IT!

We're moving on to Part Two...

Part Two
Now You Don't!
(Ways to 'release' it!)

What To Do!

This is where almost everyone

gets it **wrong!**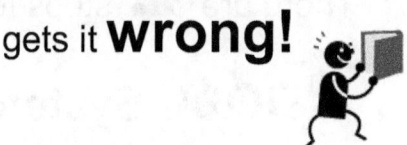

Because you're reading this book...

you'll know the

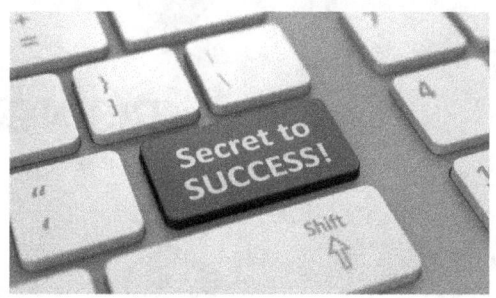

What you are about to learn is my *secret*

DO*60* System™

- ➤ It ***doesn't take*** a lot of ***time***!
- ➤ It will work for ***everyone***!
- ➤ It can be used ***everywhere***!

There are **2** steps to the

DO*60* System™

Step 1 -

the level from **RISING!**

Step 2 -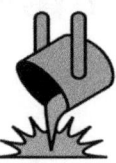

RELEASE so the level drops!

Each step must be done *in order...*

Step 1 ➡ Step 2

Each step must be done *for 60 Secs.*

Just so this makes sense…

In order to 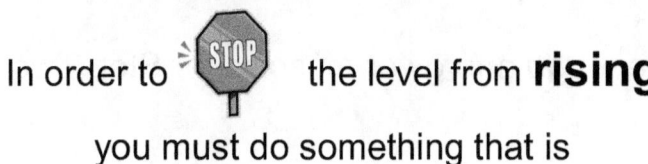 the level from **rising** you must do something that is

calming for you!

Calming = Activities that require

NO energy or muscles

be used!

I'm afraid I have a little bit of

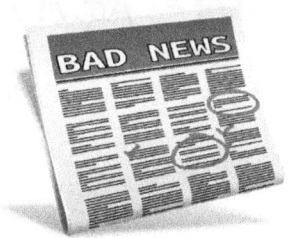

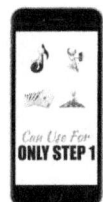 You can **ONLY** use your cell phone for this first step!

Cell phones **_DO NOT_** require

enough energy or muscles for Step Two.

Now,

In order to 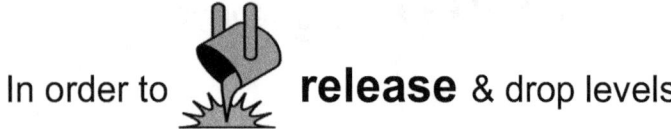 **release** & drop levels

you must do something _you like_

that is ACTIVE

Active = Activities that **DO** require

energy & muscles

BE USED!

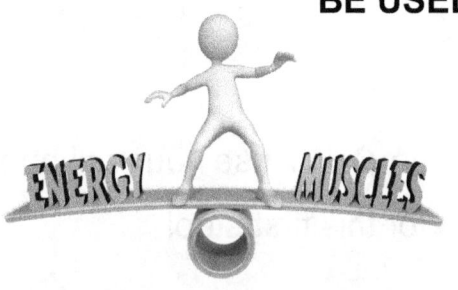

So let's apply this to our stress bottle…

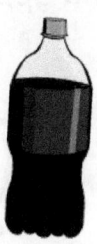

Step 1 -  **the pressure**

from continuing to build up!

Step 2 - 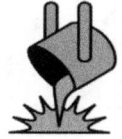 **the pressure**

that's been built up inside!

Each step:

✓ Must be done **in order**

✓ Must be done for **60 secs.**

** Otherwise the system won't work **40

And applied to our stress tub…

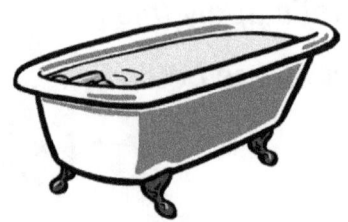

Step 1 -  **the level**

from continuing to rise!

Step 2 - 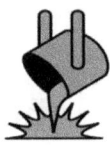 **the level**

that's been raised already!

Where most people get it wrong…

They only *turn OFF the water.*

They **DON'T** do Step 2 - RELEASE!

How To Do It!
Step 1

Sign Up Today!

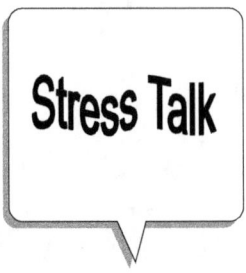

This 5-minute video newsletter will give you more tips, tools, & rules for taking control of…

STRESS!

Sign up at:

StressYOUniversity.com/Stress-Talk

On the following pages are a bunch of different **"tools"**.

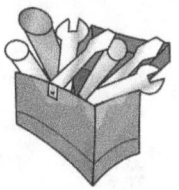

Each one is good to use for

Step 1 -

Things from **RISING!**

There are a **4 keys** to

S
  U
    C
      C
        E
          S
            S....

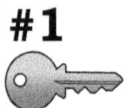 ## Try out each one.
(***even if*** you don't think it will work for you!)

 ## Do 60 Seconds.
(if you can go longer – ***do it!***
30 secs. ***is better than*** none!

 ## Keep a list.
(write down tools that end up working ***best for you***)

 ## Have more than 1!
(don't set yourself up to fail the ***more tools*** the better!)

You **must** do **Step 1** *before* Step 2

Step 1 ➡ Step 2

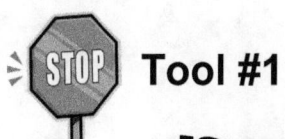 **Tool #1**

read

grab one of your favorite books

Real or **Kindle**

 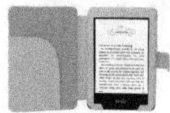

Either way….. you're reading!

 **Tool #2**

Music

Listen to one of your favorites!

Song or **Artist**

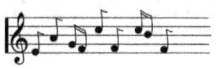 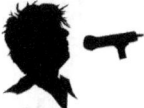

🛑 **Tool #3**

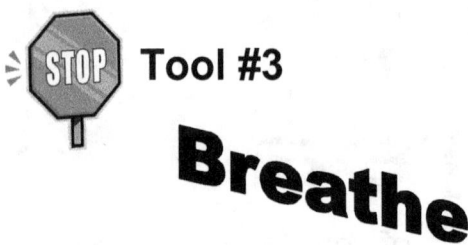

✓ **Count your breathes**

There are a couple ways to do this:

#1 **Track the # you do in 60 secs.**

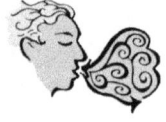

or

#2 **Set a specific # to do 10, 12, 15, 20**

Belly Breathing is best!

This gets lots of oxygen in to our brain…

Oxygen is **kryptonite** to STRESS!

Another way to *BREATHE:*

✓ Square Breathing

1) ***Breathe in*** & count to 4 in your head (1,2,3,4)

2) ***Hold it*** & count to 4 in your head (1,2,3,4)

3) ***Breathe out*** & count to 4 in your head (1,2,3,4)

4) ***Hold it*** & count to 4 in your head (1,2,3,4)

5) ***Repeat!***

Here's what it looks like!

Hold 1,2,3,4

In
1,2,3,4

Out
1,2,3,4

Hold 1,2,3,4

 **Tool #4**

Take A Time Out

Remove yourself from the situation.

Create 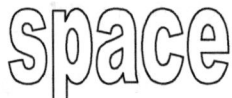 between

YOU & the situation or person

Go outside!

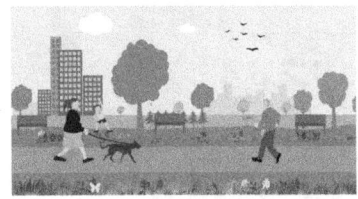

Go to another room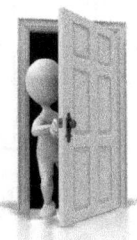

Tool #5

Mind Push Ups!

Here's how:

1. Find a quiet spot to lie down.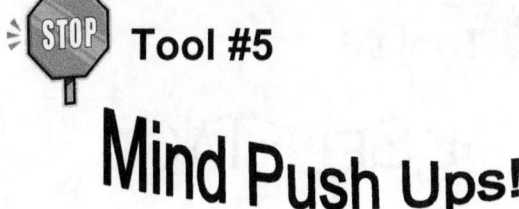

2. Set a timer for 60 secs. (*or more!*)

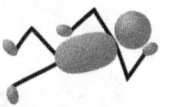

3. Put a book on your belly.

4. As you breathe in, make

 your belly & the book rise up!

5. Breathe out like your blowing candles.

6. Repeat breathes until timer goes off!

 **Tool #6**

✝ Self-Talk

Saying positive statements to yourself!

The 2 P's of Self-Talk!

1) Present

I AM…..
THIS IS….
I HAVE….

FUTURE

~~I will….~~
~~I hope…~~
~~I'm going to…~~

2) Positive

~~Don't~~ touch = TOUCH!

~~Not…~~
~~Won't…~~
~~Can't…~~

Our brain filters out the negative
& all we hear is what's after it: ***TOUCH!***

** See a list of self-talk ideas on page 69 **

 **Tool #7**

The Serenity Prayer

God,

Grant me the **serenity** to accept
 the things *I cannot change.*

The **courage** to change the things I *can.*

And the **wisdom** to know *the difference.*

Carol's
'In the Moment Serenity Prayer'

Ask yourself the following

"Can I do anything about IT

RIGHT NOW?"

If yes, ***DO it***! If NO – ***Let it go!***

Here's a few more  ***tools –***

- Guided Imagery on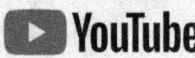

- Count to 10 **s l o w l y !**

- Watch a favorite show or movie

- Blow bubbles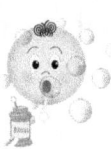

- Lie down & look at the sky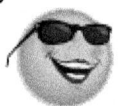

- Picture a 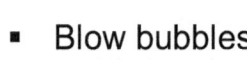 sign in your mind

- Make a "Calm Jar" Google It!

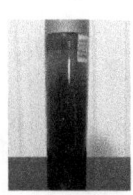

Positive Self-Talk Ideas

I no longer give power to the PAST

Today I feel peace & calm.

I am free of negative feelings.

I am learning to love myself.

Today, I choose a positive attitude.

I am terrific just the way I am!

I have all the time I need.

I am living a healthy life today

Today, I forgive all others and myself.

I am getting better one step at a time!

I am having a great day!

I am a good educator!

Can you think of other ways for you to:

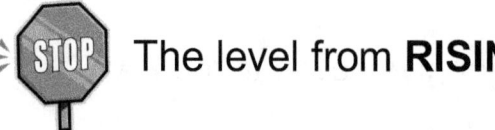 The level from **RISING!**

(Use another piece of paper if you need more room!)

Remember -

This step is one that is calming...

(Requires NO activity or muscles!)

How To Do It!
Step 2

Now we'll take a look at what to do *once* you have done

Step 1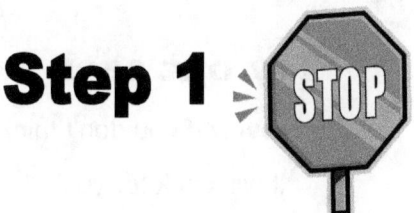

On the following pages are *more* **"tools"**…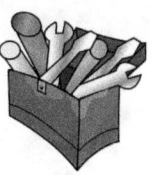

Each one of these is

good to use for

Step 2 -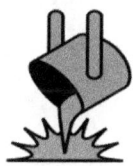

RELEASE what's there!

Again, here are those 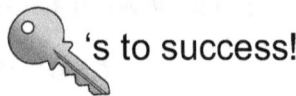's to success!

#1   Try out each one.

(***even if*** you don't think

It will work for you!)

#2   Do 60 Seconds.

(if you can go longer – ***do it!***

30 secs. ***is better than*** none!

#3   Keep a list.

(write down tools that end

up working ***best for you***)

#4   Have more than 1!

(don't set yourself up to fail

the ***more tools*** the better!)

Remember: you **must** do Step 1 ***before*** Step 2

Step 1 ⟶ Step 2

 **Tool #1**

Talk

Grab one of your favorite friends

In-person

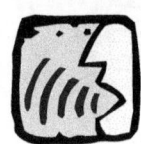

Text

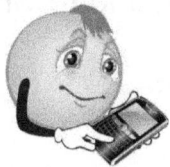

Phone

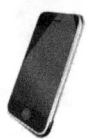

Either way….. You're *talking!*

IMPORTANT:

Talk about your *feeling*s, ***not*** the situation!

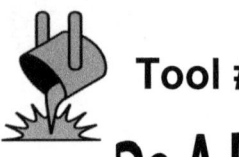 **Tool #2**

Do A Dump & Destroy

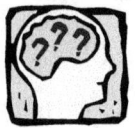

This is one of my secret weapons!

Here's what you need:
- ✓ A piece of paper
- ✓ Something to write with

1) Start writing

2) *DO NOT* READ IT

3) *Destroy IT!*

It WON'T work with a computer
It requires you to use paper!

This is different from "Journaling"....

with Dumping –

The goal = Just get it out!

Reading IT = *reloads it!*

It also works *really well* when**...

1) You can't **fall asleep** because your *mind racing*

2) You **wake up** at night & your mind is racing!

**IMPORTANT:

You must go write in *another* room for it to work.

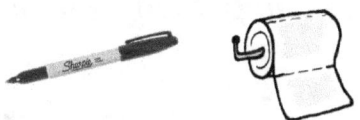

TIP: Use a sharpie & toilet paper, flush when done. No one will ever read that!

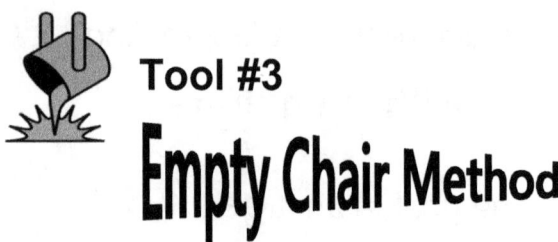

Tool #3

Empty Chair Method

When you don't have anyone

or you can't get a hold of someone

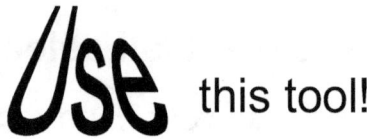 this tool!

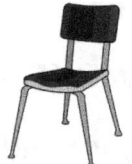

You start talking to the

"Empty Chair"

As if the person was there!

It is a great way to VENT without

getting in trouble for what you say!

Tool #4

Get ACTIVE!

There are many ways to do this!

Walk

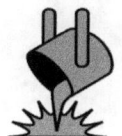

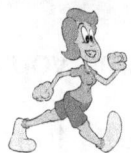

Any Kind of Exercise

Climb the Stairs

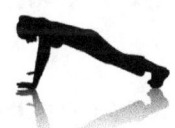

Bike

Push Ups

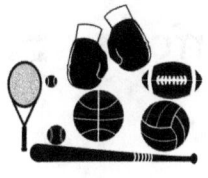

Sports

Tool #5

Music

For this tool to work, you MUST:

you **DO more** than just listen!

Dance = Any time you are *moving* to music!

 = Doesn't mean you *can*
or
KNOW the words!

Perform = Play a real **instrument**
or
AIR guitar / drums

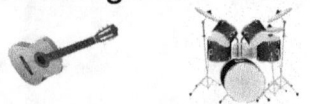

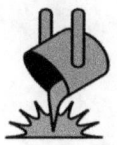 **Tool #6**

Punch n Dump!

There are **2** ways to do this:

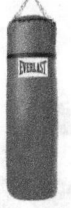

1) Use a real punching bag.

Don't have one?

You can make one using a pillow!

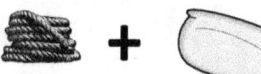

2) Air Boxing!

You must ***be sure*** to do this in a place where it is SAFE.

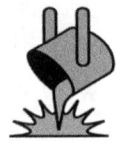 **Tool #7**

Let It Out!

When stress builds up…

Sometimes a good cry or a good laugh

is needed to ***let it out!***

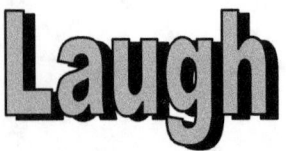 It's perfectly okay to

let the tears flow.

(Even for guys)

Watch a funny show

Try Laughter Yoga

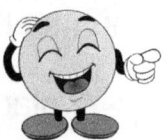

Here's a few more  tools –

- Tear up an old phone book or a bunch of paper

- Wash the car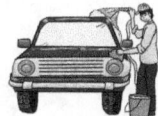

- Do some coloring!

- Clean the house!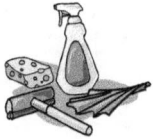

- Do some jumping jacks!

- Scream in a car or another safe place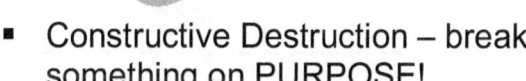

- Constructive Destruction – break something on PURPOSE!

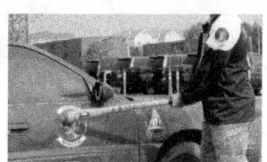

Can you think of other ways for you to:

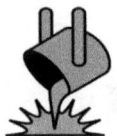 **RELEASE** what's there!

(Use another piece of paper if you need more room!)

Remember -

This step is one that is active...

(DOES require activity or muscles!)

Part Three
A Solid Foundation

In my live events – I like to see how many cars people have owned!

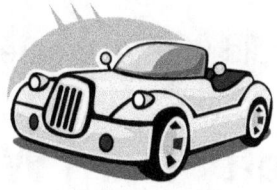

I'll ask people to raise their hands -

1

3

5

(Includes new, used, hand-me-downs, & ones that don't run anymore!)

How about you? What **number?** ___

If you've *NEVER owned a car* –
I got you covered!
I'll explain on the next page!

Now Imagine….

You had **1** car & it must last a lifetime.

How **well** would you take care of that car?!

Pretty Darn Well!

Guess what?!

    You **ARE** sitting in that **1** car -

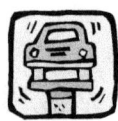 **It's called your BODY**

        &

It must last you a lifetime…

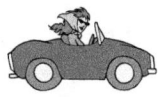

The secret to keeping your 1 **car** running?

Self-Care!

When I ask this in a live event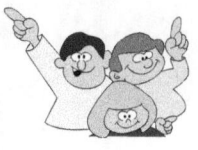
every hand goes up!

"Who already **KNOWS** that

 to *be well* you need to…

Exercise

Have good nutrition

Manage stress

Follow up w/ medical stuff?

So, what we will cover next probably

won't be 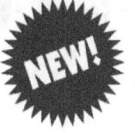 information"

Instead,

I am going to help you 👓 those

things *a little differently!*

Introducing…

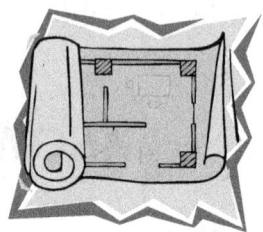

L.I.F.E
Wellness
Blueprint

I created this blueprint 25+ years ago!

I have taught to **1,000's**

in the hospitals where I've worked!

Blueprints will give you…

the ***SAME*** results every time!

Before we go any further -

I want to share my favorite Wordtool

Living

Intentionally &

Fully

Engaged!

© 2019 & licensed by Well YOUniversity, LLC
Taken from the *WordTools Series*

I need you to imagine…

    I'm standing on a 4-legged chair

        in front of you!

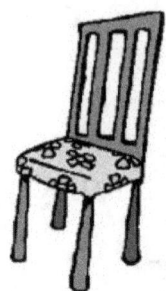

You saw off one of the legs….

    What do you think will happen?
    Do I fall on you?!

Probably not –

I have 3 legs I can still shift my weight to!

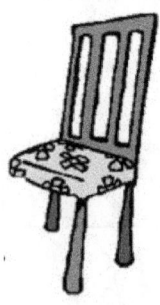

After all,

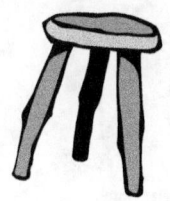 A stool only has **3 legs!**

I'll bet you've probably sat on one of these!

The problem: stools aren't too sturdy!

They tip over very easily….

You come along & saw off another leg!

What happens to me now?!

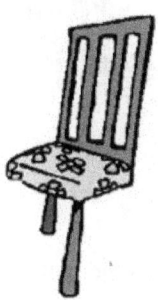

The truth is ....

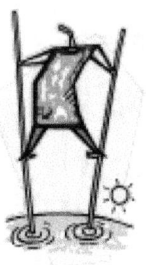

Even if I was good at stilts - it wouldn't take *much of a bump to knock me over.*

We all know

LIFE IS FULL OF **BUMPS!**

Now, you saw off the 3rd leg -

Leaving me with only **1**

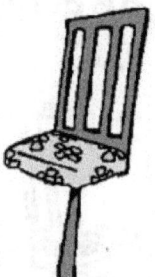

What do you think will happen to me?

You're right! I'm going down...

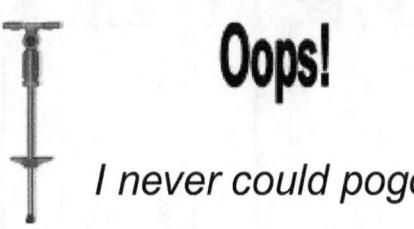

Oops!

I never could pogo stick!

So, when we expect just

Exercise or nutrition

to keep us going…..

IT CAN"T – IT IS ONLY 1 LEG!

Self Care

*(Pretty **wobbly!**)*

Building a STRONG Foundation!

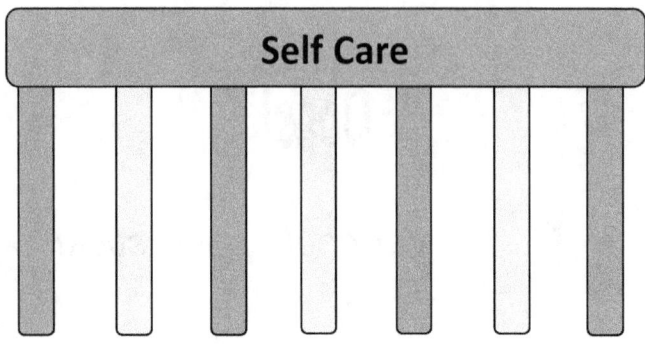

(MUCH better!)

This is what a **complete** blueprint of the foundation looks like!

Now, I want you to imagine me standing on this chair with 7 legs…

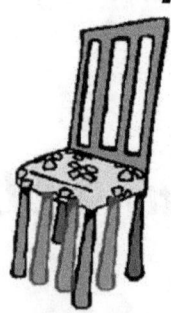

Would you agree this foundation is "**strong**", "**stable**", "**sturdy**"?

This is how your health is with the 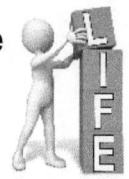 *L.I.F.E. blueprint!*

WHY

do we need to have it be so solid?

Because of this ***thing*** called STRESS!

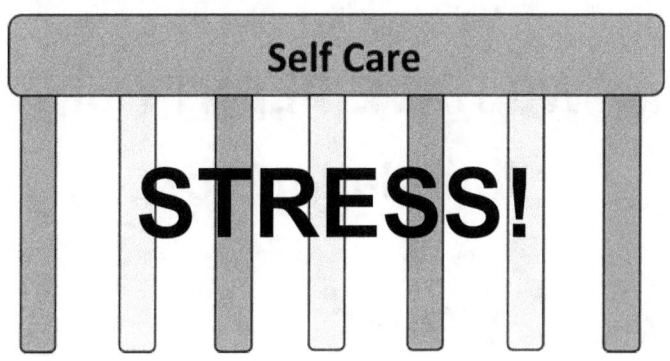

STRESS is *like an earthquake*!

It can really shake up our lives!

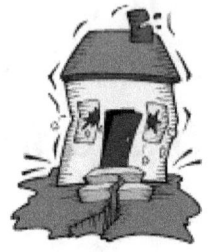

 Foundations tend to take a bruising during earthquakes & parts will fall down.

We've got to make sure

WE HAVE PLENTY of foundation so…

When we **START**

to *lose some of it,*

We've got to have enough left

to keep us **standing!**

Lost some!

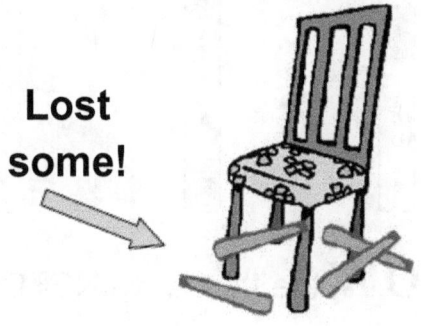

Still have some left!

Could it be that work **STRESS**

has *taken down* your **foundation?**

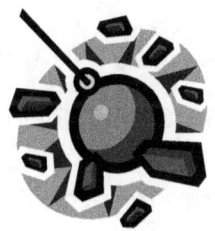

The Foundation Corners!

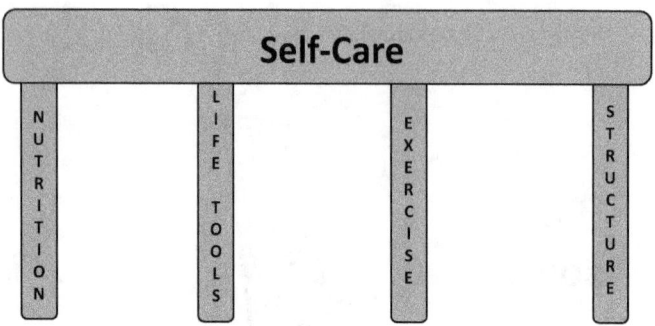

This is *how* the things we NEED:

Nutrition

        Exercise

                Life Tools

                        Structure

FIT TOGETHER!

Can you SEE why we can't just rely on exercise or nutrition alone….

It only works when

ALL 4 Foundation Corners are there!

The BIG Picture!

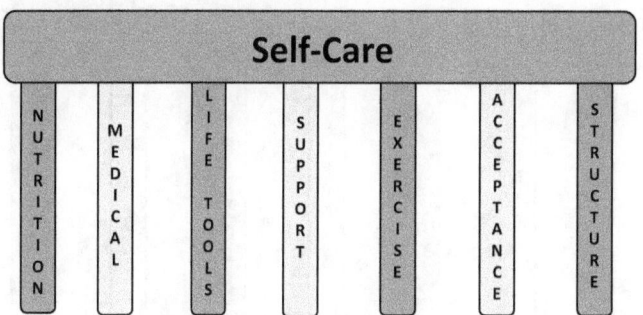

Now when we **ADD** the others –

Medical → Keep current on medical stuff!

Support → Have + people around us!

Acceptance → KNOW you need to keep doing this!

We have an even

STRONGER FOUNDATION!

I have 2 stories I'd like to share…

Self-Care						
N U T R I T I O N	M E D I C A L	L I F E T O O L S	S U P P O R T	E X E R C I S E	A C C E P T A N C E	S T R U C T U R E

This is Peter's foundation. He has a **chronic health issue** – diabetes & was *doing well* for the past **5 years.**

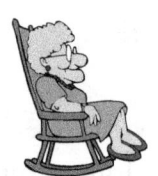

He suddenly became the **Primary caregiver** for his elderly parents.

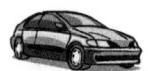

This meant every day he had to drive **45** miles one-way to get to their house.

When they started needing more help,
Peter's life was turned 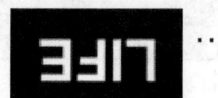 ......

So, he lost his STRUCTURE

His routine had been a solid one:

going to the gym, healthy meals,
go to his diabetes support group,
& time for playing the guitar!

He lost a **FOUNDATION CORNER:**

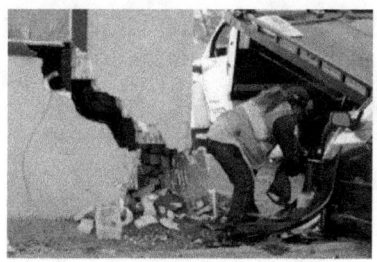

That's like losing
one corner of your house!

His self-care blueprint took a hit & became

Self-Care

| NUTRITION | MEDICAL | LIFE TOOLS | SUPPORT | EXERCISE | ACCEPTANCE |

As he needed to spend more time

at his parents, he lost another

FOUNDATION CORNER:

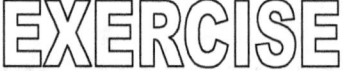

So now his self-care looked like this:

Self-Care

| NUTRITION | MEDICAL | LIFE TOOLS | SUPPORT | | ACCEPTANCE |

When we lose one of the 4 corners

it sets off a '***domino effect***' &

the others start to fall.

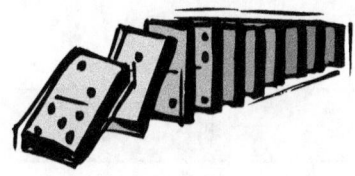

it happened quickly to Peter,
in a couple months his diabetes

was **out of control**………

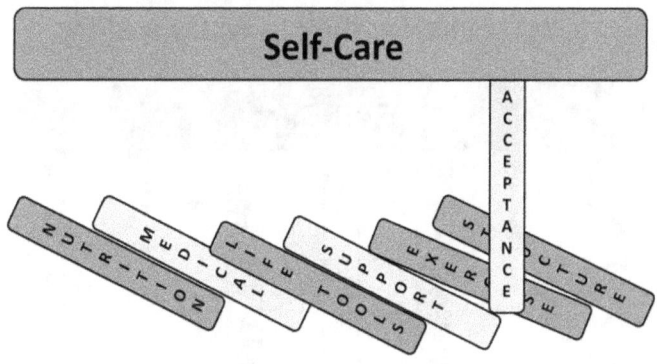

Here's what Peter's foundation looked like.

This is **_not enough_**

to keep ANYONE healthy & well!

Without his foundation... Peter ended up

Self-Care

HOSPITALIZED

The **chronic illness** he lived *with took over.*

Now I'd like to tell you Mary's story.

Self-Care						
NUTRITION	MEDICAL	LIFE TOOLS	SUPPORT	EXERCISE	ACCEPTANCE	STRUCTURE

This is her foundation.

She **has no chronic health issues.**

She's in the **best health** of her life!

Mary started a new job!
She became a case manager &
found herself working **a lot of hours.**

Too exhausted once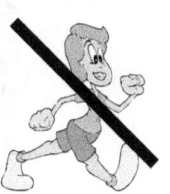
she got home, she started
missing days at her gym.

She did some walking every day at
lunchtime but this was limited to only

5 or 10 minutes

Not nearly enough to count as EXERCISE

She' used to go to the gym 6 days a week. Her workout included strength training, cardio exercise, & yoga!

She lost a **FOUNDATION CORNER:**

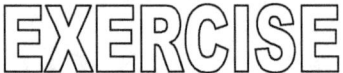

EXERCISE

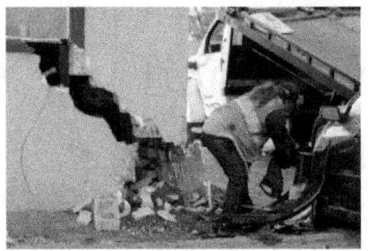

Her self-care blueprint took a hit -

Self-Care						
N U T R I T I O N	M E D I C A L	L I F E T O O L S	S U P P O R T		A C C E P T A N C E	S T R U C T U R E

As she continued to work
A LOT HOURS Mary lost another
1 ½ of her **FOUNDATION CORNERS:**

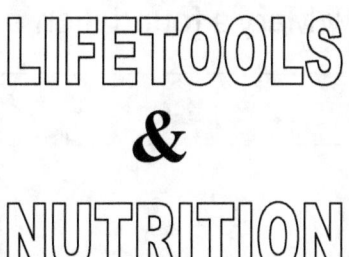

So now her self–care looked like this:

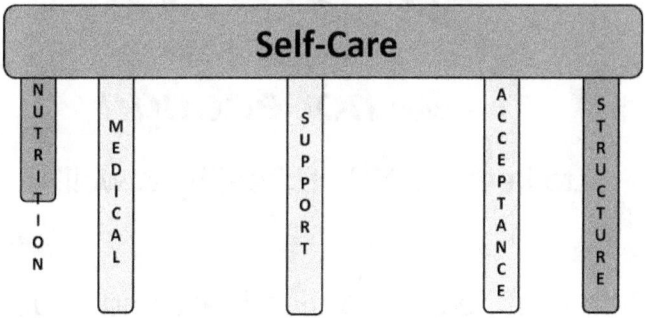

Remember the dominoes!

Lose one of the **4** foundation corners

it sets off a ***chain reaction***
& others start to fall.

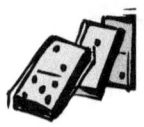 Mary's stress & work demands took its toll on her health.

Here's how Mary's foundation ended up:

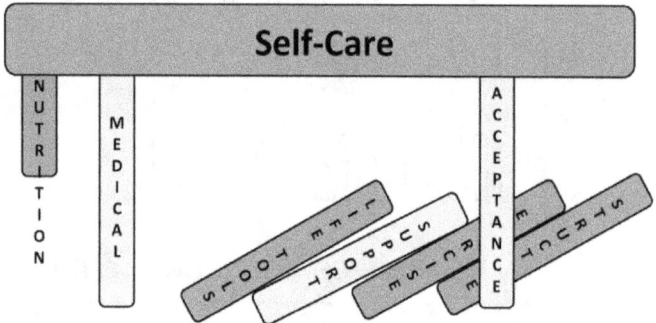

This was **_not enough_**

to keep ANYONE healthy & well!

With a limited foundation Mary ended up…

Self-Care

IN TREATMENT FOR MIGRAINES

She developed a **chronic health issue.**

The Building Process

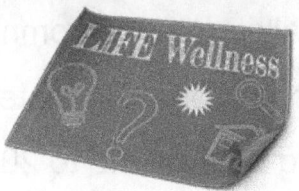

How to get started?

1) Focus on getting the FOUNDATION CORNERS in place first!

2) *START* **SMALL!**

This is the place most people get it wrong! They tend to set out to make

BIG CHANGE…..

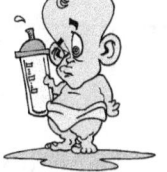

Whatever the change is –

Break it down into **baby steps**.

Let's take a 👓 at an example!

Exercise:

Start by walking during commercials.

Then go out for a 5-minute walk.

Slowly build up the time to 20-30 min.

If for some reason you

DON'T *FEEL LIKE* doing it –

Make yourself do just
1 min & then **STOP!**

This way it builds the momentum

Have you ever saved
pennies, nickels, dimes & quarters?

Then you know that small **CHANGE**
adds up to **BIG CHANGE!**

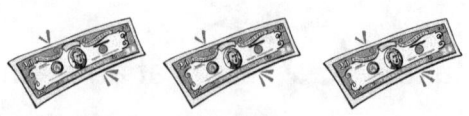

Wrap Up!

Congratulations!

You now have the "tools" to become a

Stress Master!

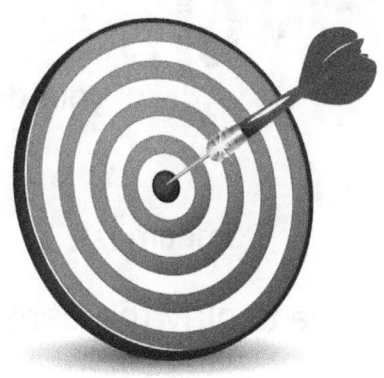

More importantly,

You can now MANAGE

your **work stress!**

It doesn't have to **RUIN**

the career you love.

You don't always get to be in

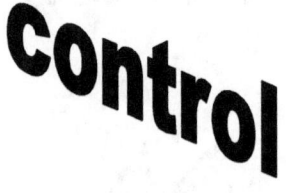

of your day...

Sometimes,

You just have to play the cards you get.

YOU

are **100% responsible** for *your response*

Part 1: Now You See It!

So,

There are **2** ways I got you to 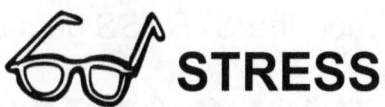 **STRESS**

Way # 1

Things happen in life that
shake a person up

And…

Just like the pressure
BUILT UP
in the bottle…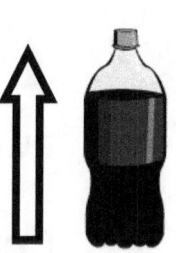

STRESS builds up *inside people!*

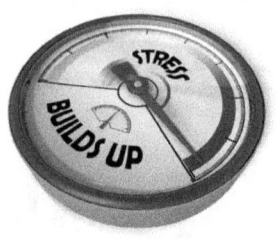

And once the *STRESS gets built up*

It stays there…

It won't go away on its own.

The **STRESS** doesn't go anywhere

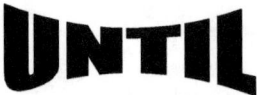

we *do something to*

Let

  It

   Out!

Way #2

People are just like a tub:

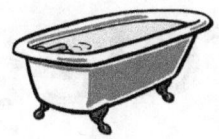

1) Your **STRESS** level starts to rise & it will keep rising until it is…

Shut off!

2) *YOU* only have *so much room* - *YOU* can only hold so much

STRESS

until *YOU* will be at

OVERFLOW!!!

And how it won't go away

until we…

release it!

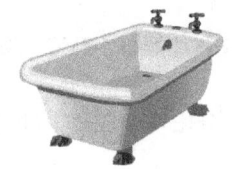

Part 2: Now You Don't!

There are **2** steps to the

DO60 System™

Step 1 -

the level from **RISING!**

Step 2 -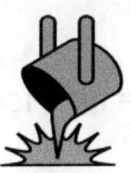

RELEASE so the level drops!

➢ **Each step** must be done *in order...*

Step 1 ⟶ Step 2

➢ **Each step** must be done *60 Secs.*

Remember:

Most everyone in the world

gets it wrong!

They don't know to DO Step 2

Now you know the secret!

Part 3

We've also looked at how easily

Stress can *ruin your health.*

The safest way to protect yourself is

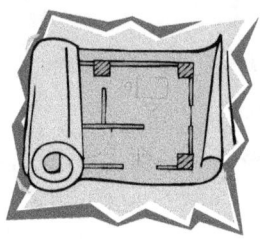

L.I.F.E
WELLNESS
BLUEPRINT

Many careers have been *taken away*

due to a person's health issues...

Bonus Tool

I created this tool for my patients & discovered I **needed** it more!

If you start ***feeling overwhelmed,*** I want you to use this:

The Serenity Prayer Stress Tool!

#1 Make a list of ALL the things that are stressing you out.

#2 Using the worksheet on the next page, place the things from your list in the appropriate section.

#1 Fold the paper on the line and **RIP IT IN HALF**. Get rid of what you CAN'T do anything about!

I have also created a couple

mini posters!

This way you can rip / cut them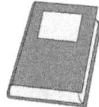
out of the book

And put them up on your fridge, computer,
or wherever you'll see them!

This will help reinforce the
new tools you're trying to
get good at using!

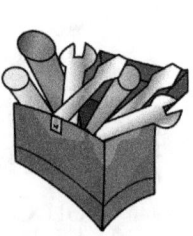

The Serenity Prayer Stress Tool!

Grant me the **serenity** to accept the things I cannot change:

_____

_____

_____

_____

- - - - - - - - - - - - - - - - - - -

The **courage** to change the things I can:

_____

_____

_____

_____

And the **wisdom** to know the difference!

Intentionally blank

DO*60* System™-

Step 1 - 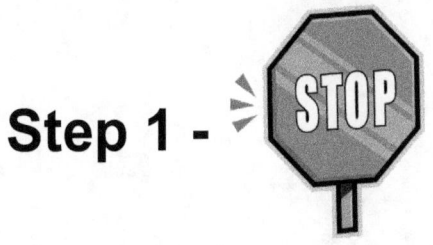   *NO* Muscles

the level from **RISING!**

Step 2 - 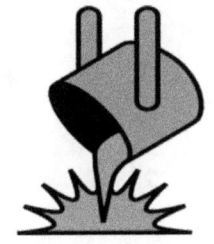   *NEEDS* Muscles

RELEASE so the level drops!

➢ **Each step** must be done *in order...*

Step 1 ⟶ Step 2

➢ **Each step** must be done *60 Secs...*

Intentionally blank

The 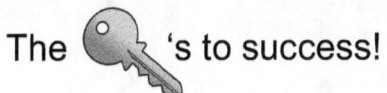's to success!

#1 Try out each one.
(***even if*** you don't think it will work for you!)

#2 Do 60 Seconds.
(if you can go longer – ***do it!*** 30 secs. ***is better than*** none!

#3 Keep a list.
(write down tools that end up working ***best for you***)

#4 Have more than 1!
(don't set yourself up to fail the ***more tools*** the better!)

The Stressometer

I find when I try to go to sleep, my mind just keeps racing about things.

   1   2   3   4   5   6   7
Not at all   All the time

I find my appetite changes, I'm either eating more or eating less.

   1   2   3   4   5   6   7
Not at all   All the time

I find myself getting really angry over the littlest things.

   1   2   3   4   5   6   7
Not at all   All the time

I find I am having increased health issues. (ie. migraines, pain, & digestive)

   1   2   3   4   5   6   7
Not at all   All the time

I find my relationship is being impacted by what goes on at work / home.

   1   2   3   4   5   6   7
Not at all   All the time

Total: _____   **Use key – page 14

Intentionally blank

Want to Speed Up Your Progress?

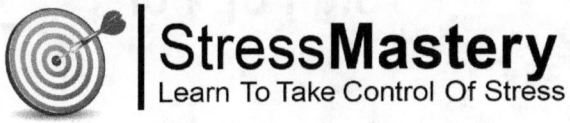

Join Carol for this

FREE

Fast Start Training!

(Sells For $297.00)

You know the **DO60**™ **System** –

Now it's time to learn the 5 keys to

being an unstoppable Stress Master!

Sign Up Now!

StressYOUniversity.com/Teachers

Sign Up For

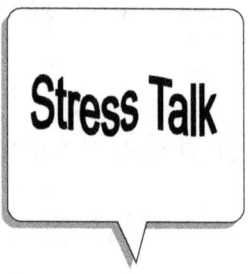

This 5 minute video newsletter will give you

more tips, tools, & rules for taking control of…

STRESS!

Sign up at:

StressYOUniversity.com/Stress-Talk

Carol's Other Resources

A Nationally Syndicated Wellness Series:

The WELL YOU Show

Mondays @ 6pm, Sundays @ 8am

Watch at: www.PrincetonTV.org

Catch past episodes at
www.TheWellYouShow.com

Want More Tools?!

Carol has written more "tool" books!

If you need help:
- ✓ Losing weight
- ✓ Dealing with anger
- ✓ Managing health issues

Take a look at the next few pages…

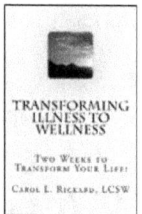 Chronic illness doesn't exclude you from having wellness. Get a blueprint to follow for taking back control of your health!

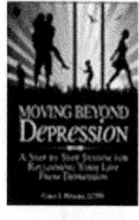 Are you sick & tired of feeling sick & tired? This is a step by step system for reclaiming your life from depression.

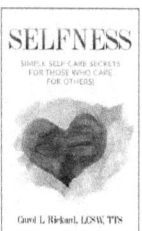 Self-care is often forgotten in this busy world. Carol offers simple and practical strategies to fit in to your busy life!

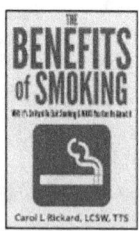 No – this is not promoting smoking! Instead, it provides the knowledge & the 'tools' to finally "Kick Cigarettes Butts"!

Available: amazon.com/author/carolrickard

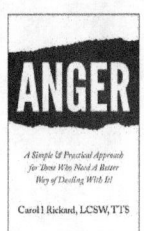

ANGER - one of the most powerful emotions there is. Learn how to manage it instead of it managing you!

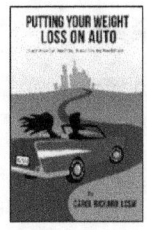

Losing weight doesn't have to be complicated! Learn the 7 *Laws of Lasting Weight Loss* a car can teach us.
Guaranteed to work!

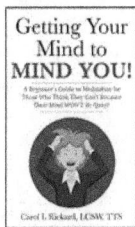

Your mind *is not* supposed to be quiet! Learn how mediation really works & change your life forever!

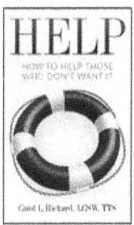

Do you find yourself struggling with what to say or how to help someone you care about? Learn how to say it & what to do!

Available: amazon.com/author/carolrickard

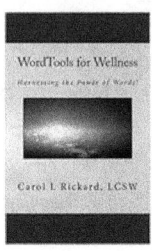

WordTools

What are words tools?
They are acronyms with purpose & meaning!

They are officially called *Artinyms™*, which is Sanskrit for "describe".

On the back of each wordtool is a question for you to answer should you choose to!

We have **4 different versions:**

Wellness Vol. 1 & 2, ***Self-Esteem*** Vol. 1 & 2
Business Vol. 1 & 2, ***Athletes*** Vol. 1

Examples:

The
Only
Day
Afforded
You!

A
Deliberate
Adjustment
Providing
Transformation

Daringly
Recognize
Experiences
As
Mine

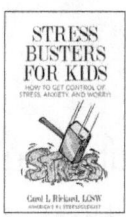

NEW RELEASE!!!!
Kid these days have to deal with so much stress. This makes sure they have the tools to succeed!!

We have three different versions of adult stress books because life circumstances can be different for each..

Choose the one that *best fits* your situation!

Caregiver

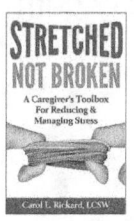

Research has shown caregivers are the MOST vulnerable. Learn quick, simple, practical tools for reducing and managing it.

Stress Eater

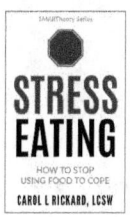

Do you find yourself eating when under stress? Get the tools & knowledge needed to break away from any old habits.

General

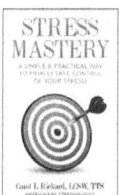

STRESS… It's all around us and NOT getting any less! Get the system Carol has taught to 1,000's & finally take control!

To Contact Carol:

Please feel free to reach out if you have questions or comments!

Email:

Carol@StressYOUniversity.com

Phone:

888 LifeTools

(543-3866)

Sign Up for Stress Talk:

CarolRickard.Tools/StressTalk

www.ingramcontent.com/pod-product-compliance
Lightning Source LLC
LaVergne TN
LVHW051838080426
835512LV00018B/2950